THE ST.ONGE
· SURVIVOR'S GUIDE

WRITTEN BY
TERRI ST. ONGE
20 Year Cancer Survivor

_me_
wishes to
you will be
next survivor.
God Bless _Terri_

Published by
TSO Company, LLC
469 Timbermill Lane
Howell, MI 48843
tstonge@att.net

ISBN: 9780615225425

Written by Terri St. Onge
Book design by Susan Pominville, Abovo Visual Communications,
Lee Lewis Walsh, Words Plus Design,
and Terri St. Onge
Logo, Cover and Section Designs by Susan Pominville,
Abovo Visual Communications
Edited by Lee Lewis Walsh, Words Plus Design

CONTENTS

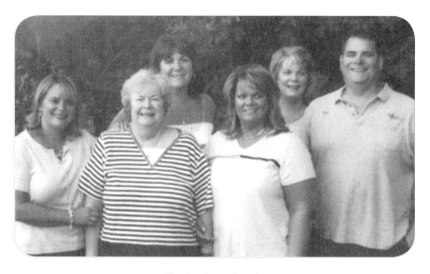

The St. Onge family
Front row: Mimi, Mom (Kathie), Sandy, Rick
Back row: Lee, Terri

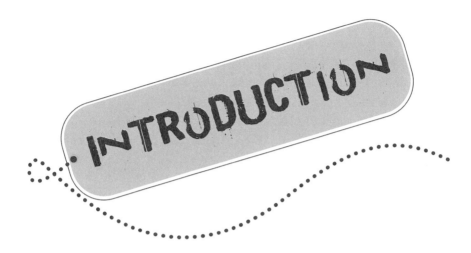

INTRODUCTION

It's hard to wrap your mind around the fact that you have breast cancer. You don't feel sick, you don't look sick. But they tell you that you're sick and everything they do to make you better... makes you sick.

I was diagnosed with breast cancer at the age of twenty-nine, and again at thirty-one. Today, in 2008, I have been a survivor for more than twenty years. My three younger sisters and my mother are also breast cancer survivors. It is my hope that sharing some of the things we learned on our roads to recovery will help others who find themselves where we once were.

Your fight against cancer will be full of overwhelming emotions and information overload for you and your family. This book is designed to help you manage your illness and your journey back to health. Keeping track of the different doctors, appointments, and tests while also trying to maintain some semblance of a normal life can seem almost impossible. I found that having one place to keep all the schedules and details, questions and answers, helps to lessen the anxiety of this very stressful situation. When you feel as if you have little or no say in your own life, being organized gives you back a sense of control.

This book is divided into easy-to-use sections: Part One gives you a place to list your doctors' contact information, the dates and outcomes of appointments, questions you want to ask (and the answers!), your prescriptions, and your medical history. Part Two includes twelve blank monthly calendars; just pencil in the dates and months when you start using this book. Part Three keeps track of that all-important resource: people who have offered to help, along with their contact information and what exactly they've offered to do for you. And Part Four offers blank pages for journaling, which can provide a beneficial outlet for your emotions during this difficult time.

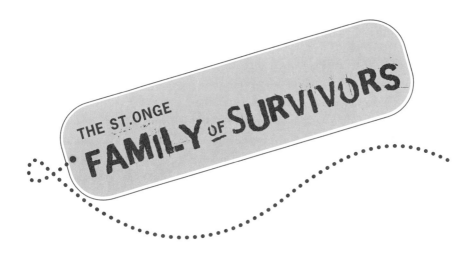

THE ST. ONGE FAMILY OF SURVIVORS

This is the story of the St. Onge women, my family of breast cancer survivors. I'm the oldest of four sisters, followed by Lee, Mimi, and Sandy. Our mother is Kathie. We also have a brother, Rick.

In 1987 I noticed a rather large and hard lump on my left breast. I really wasn't too worried since I'd had a non-malignant lump removed the previous year. On May 12, the lump was removed in the doctor's office and sent out for a biopsy. I remember the exact date because my beautiful niece Shelby was born later the same day and was even delivered by the same doctor. The following week I left work early to get my sutures removed. "Goodbye," I said, "If I have cancer I won't be back!" These were prophetic last words because when I got to the doctor's office, I was told that, at twenty-nine years of age, I had breast cancer.

I had a lumpectomy and six weeks of radiation therapy. After about two months, my life seemed to get back to normal. I checked in with my surgeon every six months for the next two years.

Five months after the two-year check-up, I thought I noticed something strange in the same breast that had been operated on — not really a lump, just a "different" feeling. My heart stopped for a second. It was weird; I could feel it sitting up but not lying down. Since my cancer I had been very careful to do breast self-exams, which was how I noticed it.

As it turned out, I had a recurrence of the same cancer. This time my course of treatment was a modified mastectomy and six months of chemotherapy. My lymph nodes came back clear. I had immediate breast reconstruction after the mastectomy. When the six months of chemo were over, I made up my mind that I was never going through that again, and so I had a prophylactic mastectomy and reconstruction. In simple terms, a prophylactic mastectomy is a surgical procedure to remove the breast before a cancer can start.

In April 2001, my youngest sister, Sandy, had an irregularity show up on her mammogram. In May it was confirmed that, at the ripe old age of thirty-two, she too had breast cancer. It was the same type of cancer I'd had: commedo carcinoma. Sandy went to the same doctors and hospital I had gone to. Because of the information gained from my experience, she decided to skip the lumpectomy and go right to more drastic surgery, a double mastectomy with a stomach tram-flap reconstruction. In June she underwent outpatient surgery to prepare the stomach muscle and tissue for the transfer to the breast area for reconstruction. In the reconstruction, which took place in July, an oval-shaped section of the stomach, including tissue and muscle, was tunneled under the skin and over the rib cage, placed through the mastectomy holes, and shaped and stitched into new breasts.

The entire family was there to see our baby sister through this ordeal. It seemed like it took forever; the surgery started at nine a.m., she got out of surgery at nine p.m., but didn't get out of recovery and up to a room of her own until eleven p.m. It was very emotional for all of us; we were tired and worried. But our sweet sister, apparently on some very good pain medication, was wheeled back into the room smiling and cracking jokes. She reassured us all with her cheerful attitude. She was also very proud of her new body parts and — still under the effects of medication — wanted to show everyone, much to the shock and embarrassment of our niece who also kept vigil at the hospital.

Sandy learned that her lymph nodes were clear, and she had an eight week convalescence period before she could return to work. With the stomach muscle pulled up to her chest, she had to stretch it in order to stand up. It was a painful process and it was almost a year before Sandy regained her strength entirely. But in July 2006 we celebrated her five-year cancer-free anniversary, a blessing for which our family is endlessly thankful. (Oh, and she has finally stopped showing off her new boobs.)

In January 2004, our sister Mimi had an irregularity show up on her mammogram, which was followed up with ultrasounds and a biopsy. At the age of forty-two, Mimi, our beautiful middle sister who had never had a serious illness or operation, was diagnosed with breast cancer. Hers was also commedo carcinoma, with early stromo invasion. Mimi's diagnosis hit the entire family hard. With me and Sandy being diagnosed at ages very young for breast cancer, it had seemed surreal, like it wasn't really happening. You get through it somehow, but it's like you're walking around in a daze — and then it's over. But with Mimi, the third of our family to be stricken, it was terrifyingly real. While Sandy and I had no children to worry about during our illness, Mimi had a husband and three young daughters to care for. Not only was she afflicted with an illness that quite possibly could take her from them, it could also be passed on to her daughters genetically. The devastation we had survived two times before had snuck up behind us and gripped our hearts.

Technology and procedures had changed since our last experience in 2001. In February 2004, Mimi had a bilateral mastectomy and a "deep inferior epigastric artery perforator flap" reconstruction. In this type of reconstruction, skin, tissue, fat, and an artery are taken from the stomach and transplanted to the mastectomy site. Her surgery lasted twelve hours with another three in recovery. Then Mimi was sent to a "step down" unit for three days immediately after her surgery. This is a step down from intensive care but allows much closer care and monitoring than in an ordinary room. It was critical that the arterial transplant be accepted so that the skin and tissue of the reconstruction survived. The temperature of the room had to be kept at eighty degrees to keep the blood vessels warm and unconstricted. Needless to say, we sweated our buns off as we tended to our sister! For Lee and me, it was another baby sister needing us and we all were fiercely protective of her those first few days.

Mimi was slower to recover her strength; she had been under anesthesia for a long time. The artery transplant was always on her mind, since she had to be so careful while it healed. Maybe because she was married or a mother, she didn't really show off her tummy tuck and chest the way Sandy had. (We just figured, "Oh well, you've seen two reconstructions, you've seen them all.") Mimi moved into a regular patient room for a few days, at which time her doctor gave her the good news that her lymph nodes were clean; the cancer had not spread. Then she came home with a hospital bed. While she was in the hospital, her friends and neighbors had organized meals for the family for the next six weeks!

Joy and happiness coursed through the whole family. Despite what many thought was bad luck, we thought we were blessed with good fortune — three sisters had survived breast cancer!

In the middle of March I decided to go ahead with my wedding to the man of my dreams. In the midst of the turmoil of 2001, I'd met a wonderful man, Dave Hammett, and was madly, deliriously happy for the first time in my life. On May 1, 2004, my dad walked his forty-six-year-old daughter down the aisle and gave me to Dave. Some say that he thought this moment might never come. (Some say neither did I!)

Our good times and happiness lasted for about four more months. Then, on September 9, 2004, we got a call saying that our beloved father, Dick St. Onge, had died in his sleep up at Lee's home in Frankfort, Michigan. I think I can truthfully say that it was the worst thing that had ever happened to all of us, including our bouts with breast cancer. The following year was one of numbness and grief. We relied on our precious mother to help us find our way back to life. She put aside her own sorrow and tended to all of our broken hearts. As a result we all clung to our mother like little children.

In October 2005, Mom called us all over to her house and broke the news that she too had had an irregular mammogram. We were stunned. She proceeded to have a biopsy and again we were shocked to hear the now-familiar news. Not only did Mom have the same cancer as the rest of us, invasive commedo carcinoma, she also had Paget's disease, an uncommon type of cancer that forms in or around the nipple. She decided to have a bilateral mastectomy with no reconstruction. We assembled at the hospital like professional family support and caregivers. I'm sure that we're an impressive if not intimidating group. We can quote medical jargon with the best of specialists. We were there to see that our mom was given the best treatment and care possible and woe to the person who slacked off!

Mom's surgery should have been routine and indeed it seemed like it went off without a hitch. But for some reason she was slow to come out of the anesthesia and get back to a room — very slow. After almost six hours in recovery, she was put in a critical care step down room and closely monitored. We finally went home around nine p.m. Then, early the next morning as each family was getting ready for work, we got a call from Mimi. The hospital phoned her around two a.m. Mom had been losing blood and her pressure was dropping slowly but steadily. If it didn't stabilize, they would be taking her back to surgery. Soon the call came telling us to run to the hospital; they were taking Mom back to the O.R. The next surgery took a very long time. We didn't find out until it was over that they'd had a hard time stopping the bleeding. Her surgeon said that they couldn't find the bleeder and so "just cauterized the hell out of it." The next four to six hours would be critical. Well, our amazingly strong, seventy-something mother pulled through and was home within two days. We weren't that surprised, because while it was becoming apparent that we had inherited an undefined breast cancer gene, we're also sure that we've inherited a very tough, "don't mess with me" gene from our mother.

Thanksgiving was both sad and happy. We missed our dad terribly, but were so grateful to have our mom with us. There are times in your life that you understand the true meaning of the Thanksgiving holiday and this was one. We were reminded that, while we had endured many losses, our blessings numbered many more.

By this time, my sister Lee had watched her sisters and mother suffer and endure and finally overcome for almost twenty years. With her doctor's support and her own conviction that she shouldn't sit back and wait for the other shoe to drop, she decided she was getting a prophylactic bilateral mastectomy. Without telling the other family members, she set up a consultation and scheduled her surgery for March 22, 2006. Lee's surgery consisted of simple mastectomies (as opposed to complete) with back-lateral tram flap reconstruction. In this procedure, tissue, skin, and muscle from one's back in the shoulder blade area is tunneled through to the mastectomy sites and constructed into breasts and even nipples.

Our family of professional supporters marched in before Lee was taken to the O.R. Big sister Terri brought her one of Dad's old T-shirts that I had washed and then left inside an old jacket of Dad's which I had never washed, so the T-shirt smelled faintly of Dad. Lee was emotional while waiting to go in to the O.R., so I brought in Dad's shirt and wrapped it around her neck and hugged her. I gave her a photo of Dad, too. I didn't know it at the time, but Lee had searched all over for her copy of that photo and was very anxious that she didn't have it. When Lee could feel our Dad's presence and could smell a faint scent like him, it calmed her and she knew everything would be fine.

Her surgery lasted about six hours and then several hours later she was put in a private room. The surgery was on Wednesday and she went home on Saturday. She said she felt pretty darned good considering that she'd just had her front removed and then her back put on her front! She went to her doctor in Grand Rapids about a week later for her first check-up. He was very happy about the surgery and she was too – she said she had the most gorgeous breasts. She would have showed them off just like Sandy had, but her lovely daughter was still not real happy with us flashing our boobs!

As the doc was changing Lee's dressing and checking the drains, he very casually said, "Oh, did you get the pathology report?" She hadn't, but she was fully expecting everything to be fine, since she had been the pro-active one. The doctor went on to say that Lee did indeed have breast cancer; it was in the lobes and her lymph nodes had hyperplasia, which is pre-cancer. Sometime in the middle of this, her ears shut down and she could hear him talking like Charlie Brown's teacher, "Blah blah blah!" Lee started shaking and crying and her husband and daughter had to be called into the exam room to calm her. The last thing we ever expected was for her to have breast cancer. It never even showed on a mammogram. Luckily she is fine now, and the doctors say that everything worked out wonderfully. Lee took a lot of grief from people who counseled her that it was wrong to have unnecessary surgery, and she did have second thoughts, but we are so thankful that she listened to her instincts and did what was right for her.

As of 2008, I am a twenty-year cancer survivor and have been cancer-free since 1990. Sandy has been a survivor since 2001, Mimi since 2004, Mom since 2005, and Lee since 2006.

So now you know a bit about me and my wonderful, crazy family of survivors. Some people think ours is a sad story, but I think it speaks of inner strength and the importance of family. We are fortunate that we are here and that we have each other. We have a special awareness that all women everywhere are sisters under our bras and T-shirts, and nothing, not even breast cancer, can mess with this special sisterhood of strength.

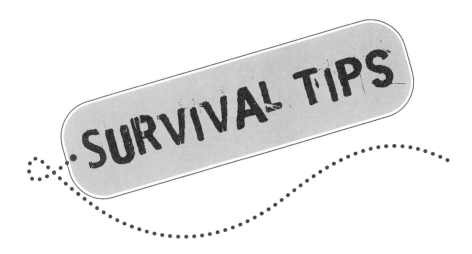

One of the hidden blessings of my family's battle against breast cancer is the knowledge we've gained. There are all kinds of things that your doctors and specialists won't think to tell you, things you wouldn't know unless you'd actually gone through the ordeal yourself. Here are a few survival tips:

• First and foremost, accept offers of help! People need to know that *you* know they care. Let them help. When this is all over, you'll pass on the help that was given you. (Trust me — passing it on becomes almost automatic.) Part Three of this book gives you a handy place to keep track of who has offered to help with what.

• People sometimes don't know *how* to help, but want to make you feel better. You'll get gifts of flowers or stuffed animals when what you really need are gas cards or groceries. It's okay to tell people what you need.

• Friends will call with offers of food, but the last thing you want is to be totally overwhelmed with people stopping by with casseroles right after you get home from the hospital. My sister Sandy drew up a meal schedule for our sister Mimi, where she listed the names of those who had offered food and assigned them a date. Having a schedule helps spread out the meals so you can actually use (and appreciate!) them.

• The time between your diagnosis and your first procedure can be particularly trying. Until you begin treatment, you may not feel like you have any control over your life, but this is normal. You can try to stay busy, or use the time to get things ready for when your treatment starts. It is important that you tell your doctor how you feel about the wait; you may be able to be moved up in the schedule.

• It's important to take control of your recovery. If you don't like a doctor or a course of treatment, don't be afraid to question him or her, or start over with someone new. At your appointments, make sure you take all the time you need to get your questions answered; don't feel rushed or that you're a bother. As questions occur to you, write them down in Part One of this book; take the book to appointments, ask the questions, and write down the answers right away.

• Do whatever it takes to be comfortable with appointments and procedures. For example, I didn't like to wear a paper gown for office exams. I didn't feel comfortable asking questions with a "paper towel" clutched to my chest and, besides, it was cold while I waited. So I began to bring a robe with me to appointments, or I would stop at the X-ray department to get a gown. Once I had on a nice warm robe or gown, I pulled out my list and questioned away. My surgeon began to ask, "Do you have your list?"

• When you go to the hospital or to an appointment, make sure that you're "doctor dressed," in easy-on, easy-off clothing with no jewelry. Buttoned shirts are much easier to slip on after X-rays or radiation, and so are pull-on, loose-fitting pants. (Plus, after a day of pulling a shirt on and off over your head, imagine what your hair will look like!)

• While you're in the hospital, remember that the "squeaky" patient gets the "grease." Ask the caregivers for what you need. You're not bothering them! Taking care of you is their job and they won't get mad if you ask them for something.

• Many people don't realize that you can have someone stay in your hospital room 24/7. It can be very comforting and also very helpful to have a family member or friend stay with you through the days and nights following surgery. When the nurses are busy, you have someone right there to get you a cool cloth or feed you ice chips or help you to the bathroom. We made a twenty-four hour schedule and took turns. Even our brother Rick helped out.

• For hospital wear, I like buttoned pajama tops and pull-on pants rather than nightgowns. That way, when the doctor or nurse examines you, your whole body doesn't have to be exposed; at a time when everyone is poking and prodding you, it's important to preserve some sense of dignity. I also recommend short, zip-up fleece jackets or bed jackets. They are more comfortable in bed than full-length robes, yet they're warm and you're covered up when visitors come to see you. I also take thick, warm socks with me to the hospital and keep them on in bed, and then I don't have to put on slippers to get up.

• My sister Lee made me two small pink fleece pillows, crescent-shaped and only about a foot long. They're great to tuck under a sore arm or at the small of your back and they really helped make me much more comfortable.

• Sometimes after surgery you go home with "drains" — tubes stuck into your body connected to a bottle that is pinned to your clothing. They are both hard to hide and hard to shower with: where do you pin them when you're naked? My sister Mimi came up with the idea of using a lanyard. Hang it around your neck and clip the pins on it while you shower. When I was going out or working, I would put my drain bottles in a fanny pack at my waist to hide them.

• It can take a long time to fully recover your strength and stamina after surgery and treatment. It's not unusual to take a full year before you feel back to normal. Take the time to let yourself heal inside and out. If you find yourself tiring easily, take a nap. Don't worry; you will feel better — it just takes time.

• Ask your doctor to send you to physical therapy. A few weeks of rehabilitation can do wonders to recover mobility and strength in wounded muscle and tissue. It can also help to limit scar tissue from forming.

• I drank lemonade after chemotherapy and anesthesia to help flush the "junk" out of my body. It had to be the frozen concentrate with pulp in it. I don't know why but it made me feel better; it settled my stomach and gave me electrolytes. Others also agree that lemonade helps them feel better faster after surgery and chemo.

• Although it may sound trite, vanity plays a big part in your recovery. It's very hard to feel like crap every day and then to look like crap also. It's normal to feel bad about how you look! Your hair falls out, you gain or lose weight, something is cut out or off, and then they tell you, "You're okay now. You're lucky!" You get this body back you don't even recognize as your own and you think "Lucky?!" But it's normal. Allow yourself to grieve for all your losses; don't try to suppress it. The sooner you feel *as bad as you're going to*, the sooner you can start to recover.

• Find something to cherish in every single day. A few years ago, my dad called me and said he was making pies and forgot to get something; could I please bring some over? It was about eight p.m. and I was beat but I said, "Sure, no problem." Someone later told me, "I can't believe you ran over to your Dad at eight at night!" I looked at her and just smiled. I always knew that there would come a day when I would give anything to run over to see my dad. When he died, I remembered how we finished making the pies together and we laughed and talked. That errand ended up being a gift I gave myself and I cherish that memory.

• Be happy every day and let it show. Try to make others happy. Find happiness in someone else's joy. Do nice things for no reason. Even on days when you feel like crap, *acting* happy will make you feel better. And pretty soon it will no longer be just acting.

• Your battle against cancer will be the longest, shortest time in your life. At first it seems like treatment will take forever, and then you think, "It's been three months already?" Remember: you can't control the outcome, but you can control the journey.

There were days when I wondered if I'd make it and days when I wondered if I even wanted to. But I did make it, and so did my mother and my sisters — and so can you. My life with cancer has made me tougher and able to see things more clearly. It's really true — what doesn't kill you makes you stronger.

PART ONE

DOCS, PRESCRIPTIONS & MEDICAL HISTORY

attach business card here

Doctor _____

Specialty _____

Call this doctor if I am having trouble with _____

_____

Phone _____

After hours phone _____

Staff names _____

Address _____

Directions _____

_____

Prescriptions _____

_____

A good laugh and a long sleep are the best cures in the doctor's book.
— Irish Proverb

Appointment   Questions
Date/Time   & Answers

_____

_____

_____

_____

_____

_____

_____

_____

_____

_____

_____

_____

_____

Appointment Date/Time	Questions & Answers

DOCTORS

Doctor _____

Specialty _____

Call this doctor if I am having trouble with _____

_____

Phone _____

After hours phone _____

Staff names _____

Address _____

Directions _____

_____

Prescriptions _____

_____

Appointment Date/Time	Questions & Answers

Appointment Date/Time	Questions & Answers

attach business card here

Doctor _____

Specialty _____

Call this doctor if I am having trouble with _____

_____

Phone _____

After hours phone _____

Staff names _____

Address _____

Directions _____

_____

Prescriptions _____

_____

Appointment   Questions
Date/Time   & Answers

Appointment Date/Time	Questions & Answers

attach business card here

Doctor _____

Specialty _____

Call this doctor if I am having trouble with _____

_____

Phone _____

After hours phone _____

Staff names _____

Address _____

Directions _____

_____

Prescriptions _____

_____

Appointment Date/Time	Questions & Answers

Appointment
Date/Time

Questions
& Answers

_____

_____

_____

_____

_____

_____

_____

_____

_____

_____

_____

_____

_____

```
┌ ─ ─ ─ ─ ─ ─ ─ ─ ─ ─ ─ ─ ─ ─ ─ ┐
│                               │
│                               │
│                               │
│       attach business card here      │
│                               │
│                               │
│                               │
└ ─ ─ ─ ─ ─ ─ ─ ─ ─ ─ ─ ─ ─ ─ ─ ┘
```

Doctor _____

Specialty _____

Call this doctor if I am having trouble with _____

_____

Phone _____

After hours phone _____

Staff names _____

Address _____

Directions _____

_____

Prescriptions _____

_____

Appointment   Questions
Date/Time   & Answers

_____

_____

_____

_____

_____

_____

_____

_____

_____

_____

_____

DOCTORS

Appointment Date/Time	Questions & Answers

DOCTORS

Doctor _____

Specialty _____

Call this doctor if I am having trouble with _____

_____

Phone _____

After hours phone _____

Staff names _____

Address _____

Directions _____

_____

Prescriptions _____

_____

Appointment Date/Time	Questions & Answers

Appointment Date/Time	Questions & Answers

attach business card here

Doctor _____

Specialty _____

Call this doctor if I am having trouble with _____

_____

Phone _____

After hours phone _____

Staff names _____

Address _____

Directions _____

_____

Prescriptions _____

_____

Appointment Date/Time	Questions & Answers

DOCTORS

Appointment
Date/Time

Questions
& Answers

DOCTORS

attach business card here

DOCTORS

Doctor ____________________

Specialty ____________________

Call this doctor if I am having trouble with ____________________

____

Phone ____________________

After hours phone ____________________

Staff names ____________________

Address ____________________

Directions ____________________

____

Prescriptions ____________________

____

Appointment Date/Time	Questions & Answers

Appointment Date/Time	Questions & Answers

attach business card here

Doctor _____

Specialty _____

Call this doctor if I am having trouble with _____

_____

Phone _____

After hours phone _____

Staff names _____

Address _____

Directions _____

_____

Prescriptions _____

_____

Appointment   Questions
Date/Time   & Answers

_____

_____

_____

_____

_____

_____

_____

_____

_____

_____

_____

_____

Appointment Date/Time	Questions & Answers

attach business card here

Doctor _____

Specialty _____

Call this doctor if I am having trouble with _____

_____

Phone _____

After hours phone _____

Staff names _____

Address _____

Directions _____

_____

Prescriptions _____

_____

Appointment Date/Time	Questions & Answers

Appointment Date/Time	Questions & Answers

Notes

Insurance company _____

Phone _____

Contract numbers _____

Co-pay info _____

Drug allergies _____

_____

Blood type _____

Drug name _____ Dose _____

Purpose _____

Doctor name _____ Phone _____

Pharmacy name _____ Phone _____

Address _____

Hours _____

Other info _____

Drug name _____ Dose _____

Purpose _____

Doctor name _____ Phone _____

Pharmacy name _____ Phone _____

Address _____

Hours _____

Other info _____

_____

Drug name _____ Dose _____

Purpose _____

Doctor name _____ Phone _____

Pharmacy name _____ Phone _____

Address _____

Hours _____

Other info _____

_____

Drug name _____ Dose _____

Purpose _____

Doctor name _____ Phone _____

Pharmacy name _____ Phone _____

Address _____

Hours _____

Other info _____

_____

Drug name _____ Dose _____

Purpose _____

Doctor name _____ Phone _____

Pharmacy name _____ Phone _____

Address _____

Hours _____

Other info _____

_____

Drug name _____ Dose _____

Purpose _____

Doctor name _____ Phone _____

Pharmacy name _____ Phone _____

Address _____

Hours _____

Other info _____

_____

Drug name _____ Dose _____

Purpose _____

Doctor name _____ Phone _____

Pharmacy name _____ Phone _____

Address _____

Hours _____

Other info _____

_____

Drug name _____ Dose _____

Purpose _____

Doctor name _____ Phone _____

Pharmacy name _____ Phone _____

Address _____

Hours _____

Other info _____

_____

Drug name _____ Dose _____

Purpose _____

Doctor name _____ Phone _____

Pharmacy name _____ Phone _____

Address _____

Hours _____

Other info _____

_____

Drug name _____ Dose _____

Purpose _____

Doctor name _____ Phone _____

Pharmacy name _____ Phone _____

Address _____

Hours _____

Other info _____

_____

Drug name _____ Dose _____

Purpose _____

Doctor name _____ Phone _____

Pharmacy name _____ Phone _____

Address _____

Hours _____

Other info _____

_____

Drug name _____ Dose _____

Purpose _____

Doctor name _____ Phone _____

Pharmacy name _____ Phone _____

Address _____

Hours _____

Other info _____

_____

Drug name _____ Dose _____

Purpose _____

Doctor name _____ Phone _____

Pharmacy name _____ Phone _____

Address _____

Hours _____

Other info _____

_____

Drug name _____ Dose _____

Purpose _____

Doctor name _____ Phone _____

Pharmacy name _____ Phone _____

Address _____

Hours _____

Other info _____

_____

Drug name _____ Dose _____

Purpose _____

Doctor name _____ Phone _____

Pharmacy name _____ Phone _____

Address _____

Hours _____

Other info _____

_____

Drug name _____ Dose _____

Purpose _____

Doctor name _____ Phone _____

Pharmacy name _____ Phone _____

Address _____

Hours _____

Other info _____

_____

Drug name _____ Dose _____

Purpose _____

Doctor name _____ Phone _____

Pharmacy name _____ Phone _____

Address _____

Hours _____

Other info _____

_____

Drug name _____ Dose _____

Purpose _____

Doctor name _____ Phone _____

Pharmacy name _____ Phone _____

Address _____

Hours _____

Other info _____

_____

Drug name _____ Dose _____

Purpose _____

Doctor name _____ Phone _____

Pharmacy name _____ Phone _____

Address _____

Hours _____

Other info _____

_____

Drug name ————————————— Dose ————————————

Purpose ——————————————————————————

Doctor name ——————————— Phone ————————————

Pharmacy name ——————————— Phone ————————————

Address ——————————————————————————

Hours ——————————————————————————

Other info ——————————————————————————

—————————————————————————————

Drug name ————————————— Dose ————————————

Purpose ——————————————————————————

Doctor name ——————————— Phone ————————————

Pharmacy name ——————————— Phone ————————————

Address ——————————————————————————

Hours ——————————————————————————

Other info ——————————————————————————

—————————————————————————————

Drug name _____ Dose _____

Purpose _____

Doctor name _____ Phone _____

Pharmacy name _____ Phone _____

Address _____

Hours _____

Other info _____

_____

Drug name _____ Dose _____

Purpose _____

Doctor name _____ Phone _____

Pharmacy name _____ Phone _____

Address _____

Hours _____

Other info _____

_____

Surgeries

Dates

Medical Conditions or Illnesses   Dates

_____

_____

_____

_____

_____

_____

_____

_____

_____

_____

Joint Replacements/Implants _____

_____

_____

_____

Removable Dental Work _____

_____

_____

_____

Other _____

_____

_____

_____

_____

MEDICAL HISTORY

MEDICAL HISTORY

Other _____

_____

_____

_____

_____

_____

_____

_____

_____

_____

_____

_____

PART TWO

CALENDAR

Sunday	Monday	Tuesday	Wednesday

CALENDAR

With each passing day, I didn't lose hope. I fought to have more.
— Amy Tan, One Hundred Secret Senses

Thursday	Friday	Saturday	NOTES

Sunday	Monday	Tuesday	Wednesday

CALENDAR

Aerodynamically, the bumble bee shouldn't be able to fly, but the bumble bee doesn't know it so it goes on flying anyway. — Mary Kay Ash

Thursday	Friday	Saturday	NOTES

MONTH: _____

Sunday	Monday	Tuesday	Wednesday

CALENDAR

All of us, at certain moments of our lives, need to take advice and to
receive help from other people. — Alexis Carrel

Thursday	Friday	Saturday	NOTES

Sunday	Monday	Tuesday	Wednesday

CALENDAR

It's hard to beat a person who never gives up.
— Babe Ruth

Thursday	Friday	Saturday	NOTES

Sunday	Monday	Tuesday	Wednesday

CALENDAR

I am a little deaf, a little blind, a little impotent, and on top of this are two or three abominable infirmities, but nothing destroys my hope. — *Voltaire*

Thursday	Friday	Saturday	NOTES

MONTH: _____

Sunday	Monday	Tuesday	Wednesday

We are like tea bags: we don't know our own strength until we're in hot water.
— Sister Busche

Thursday	Friday	Saturday	NOTES

CALENDAR

MONTH: _____

Sunday	Monday	Tuesday	Wednesday

CALENDAR

Thursday	Friday	Saturday	NOTES

CALENDAR

MONTH: _____

Sunday	Monday	Tuesday	Wednesday

CALENDAR

Most of the important things in the world have been accomplished by people who have kept on trying when there seemed to be no hope at all. — Dale Carnegie

Thursday	Friday	Saturday	NOTES

CALENDAR

Sunday	Monday	Tuesday	Wednesday

CALENDAR

Write it on your heart that every day is the best day of the year.
— Ralph Waldo Emerson

Thursday	Friday	Saturday	NOTES

Sunday	Monday	Tuesday	Wednesday

CALENDAR

Laughter rises out of tragedy, when you need it the most, and
rewards you for your courage. — *Erma Bombeck*

Thursday	Friday	Saturday	NOTES

Sunday	Monday	Tuesday	Wednesday

CALENDAR

Be kind, for everyone you meet is fighting a hard battle.
— Plato

Thursday	Friday	Saturday	NOTES

MONTH: _____

Sunday	Monday	Tuesday	Wednesday

For every soul, there is a guardian watching it.
— The Koran

Thursday	Friday	Saturday	NOTES

CALENDAR

2009

JANUARY
S	M	T	W	T	F	S
				1	2	3
4	5	6	7	8	9	10
11	12	13	14	15	16	17
18	19	20	21	22	23	24
25	26	27	28	29	30	31

FEBRUARY
S	M	T	W	T	F	S
1	2	3	4	5	6	7
8	9	10	11	12	13	14
15	16	17	18	19	20	21
22	23	24	25	26	27	28

MARCH
S	M	T	W	T	F	S
1	2	3	4	5	6	7
8	9	10	11	12	13	14
15	16	17	18	19	20	21
22	23	24	25	26	27	28
29	30	31				

APRIL
S	M	T	W	T	F	S
			1	2	3	4
5	6	7	8	9	10	11
12	13	14	15	16	17	18
19	20	21	22	23	24	25
26	27	28	29	30		

MAY
S	M	T	W	T	F	S
					1	2
3	4	5	6	7	8	9
10	11	12	13	14	15	16
17	18	19	20	21	22	23
24/31	25	26	27	28	29	30

JUNE
S	M	T	W	T	F	S
	1	2	3	4	5	6
7	8	9	10	11	12	13
14	15	16	17	18	19	20
21	22	23	24	25	26	27
28	29	30				

JULY
S	M	T	W	T	F	S
			1	2	3	4
5	6	7	8	9	10	11
12	13	14	15	16	17	18
19	20	21	22	23	24	25
26	27	28	29	30	31	

AUGUST
S	M	T	W	T	F	S
						1
2	3	4	5	6	7	8
9	10	11	12	13	14	15
16	17	18	19	20	21	22
23/30	24/31	25	26	27	28	29

SEPTEMBER
S	M	T	W	T	F	S
		1	2	3	4	5
6	7	8	9	10	11	12
13	14	15	16	17	18	19
20	21	22	23	24	25	26
27	28	29	30			

OCTOBER
S	M	T	W	T	F	S
				1	2	3
4	5	6	7	8	9	10
11	12	13	14	15	16	17
18	19	20	21	22	23	24
25	26	27	28	29	30	31

NOVEMBER
S	M	T	W	T	F	S
1	2	3	4	5	6	7
8	9	10	11	12	13	14
15	16	17	18	19	20	21
22	23	24	25	26	27	28
29	30					

DECEMBER
S	M	T	W	T	F	S
		1	2	3	4	5
6	7	8	9	10	11	12
13	14	15	16	17	18	19
20	21	22	23	24	25	26
27	28	29	30	31		

2010

JANUARY
S	M	T	W	T	F	S
					1	2
3	4	5	6	7	8	9
10	11	12	13	14	15	16
17	18	19	20	21	22	23
24/31	25	26	27	28	29	30

FEBRUARY
S	M	T	W	T	F	S
	1	2	3	4	5	6
7	8	9	10	11	12	13
14	15	16	17	18	19	20
21	22	23	24	25	26	27
28						

MARCH
S	M	T	W	T	F	S
	1	2	3	4	5	6
7	8	9	10	11	12	13
14	15	16	17	18	19	20
21	22	23	24	25	26	27
28	29	30	31			

APRIL
S	M	T	W	T	F	S
				1	2	3
4	5	6	7	8	9	10
11	12	13	14	15	16	17
18	19	20	21	22	23	24
25	26	27	28	29	30	

MAY
S	M	T	W	T	F	S
						1
2	3	4	5	6	7	8
9	10	11	12	13	14	15
16	17	18	19	20	21	22
23/30	24/31	25	26	27	28	29

JUNE
S	M	T	W	T	F	S
		1	2	3	4	5
6	7	8	9	10	11	12
13	14	15	16	17	18	19
20	21	22	23	24	25	26
27	28	29	30			

JULY
S	M	T	W	T	F	S
				1	2	3
4	5	6	7	8	9	10
11	12	13	14	15	16	17
18	19	20	21	22	23	24
25	26	27	28	29	30	31

AUGUST
S	M	T	W	T	F	S
1	2	3	4	5	6	7
8	9	10	11	12	13	14
15	16	17	18	19	20	21
22	23	24	25	26	27	28
29	30	31				

SEPTEMBER
S	M	T	W	T	F	S
			1	2	3	4
5	6	7	8	9	10	11
12	13	14	15	16	17	18
19	20	21	22	23	24	25
26	27	28	29	30		

OCTOBER
S	M	T	W	T	F	S
					1	2
3	4	5	6	7	8	9
10	11	12	13	14	15	16
17	18	19	20	21	22	23
24/31	25	26	27	28	29	30

NOVEMBER
S	M	T	W	T	F	S
	1	2	3	4	5	6
7	8	9	10	11	12	13
14	15	16	17	18	19	20
21	22	23	24	25	26	27
28	29	30				

DECEMBER
S	M	T	W	T	F	S
			1	2	3	4
5	6	7	8	9	10	11
12	13	14	15	16	17	18
19	20	21	22	23	24	25
26	27	28	29	30	31	

2011

JANUARY
S	M	T	W	T	F	S
						1
2	3	4	5	6	7	8
9	10	11	12	13	14	15
16	17	18	19	20	21	22
23/30	24/31	25	26	27	28	29

FEBRUARY
S	M	T	W	T	F	S
		1	2	3	4	5
6	7	8	9	10	11	12
13	14	15	16	17	18	19
20	21	22	23	24	25	26
27	28					

MARCH
S	M	T	W	T	F	S
		1	2	3	4	5
6	7	8	9	10	11	12
13	14	15	16	17	18	19
20	21	22	23	24	25	26
27	28	29	30	31		

APRIL
S	M	T	W	T	F	S
					1	2
3	4	5	6	7	8	9
10	11	12	13	14	15	16
17	18	19	20	21	22	23
24	25	26	27	28	29	30

MAY
S	M	T	W	T	F	S
1	2	3	4	5	6	7
8	9	10	11	12	13	14
15	16	17	18	19	20	21
22	23	24	25	26	27	28
29	30	31				

JUNE
S	M	T	W	T	F	S
			1	2	3	4
5	6	7	8	9	10	11
12	13	14	15	16	17	18
19	20	21	22	23	24	25
26	27	28	29	30		

JULY
S	M	T	W	T	F	S
					1	2
3	4	5	6	7	8	9
10	11	12	13	14	15	16
17	18	19	20	21	22	23
24/31	25	26	27	28	29	30

AUGUST
S	M	T	W	T	F	S
	1	2	3	4	5	6
7	8	9	10	11	12	13
14	15	16	17	18	19	20
21	22	23	24	25	26	27
28	29	30	31			

SEPTEMBER
S	M	T	W	T	F	S
				1	2	3
4	5	6	7	8	9	10
11	12	13	14	15	16	17
18	19	20	21	22	23	24
25	26	27	28	29	30	

OCTOBER
S	M	T	W	T	F	S
						1
2	3	4	5	6	7	8
9	10	11	12	13	14	15
16	17	18	19	20	21	22
23/30	24/31	25	26	27	28	29

NOVEMBER
S	M	T	W	T	F	S
		1	2	3	4	5
6	7	8	9	10	11	12
13	14	15	16	17	18	19
20	21	22	23	24	25	26
27	28	29	30			

DECEMBER
S	M	T	W	T	F	S
				1	2	3
4	5	6	7	8	9	10
11	12	13	14	15	16	17
18	19	20	21	22	23	24
25	26	27	28	29	30	31

In the depth of winter, I finally learned that there was within me
an invincible summer. — Albert Camus

Notes

Notes

Notes

Notes

Notes

Notes

Notes

Notes

Notes

Notes

PART THREE

CALL ME IF YOU NEED ANYTHING...

If there's anything I can do. . .

Name _____

Address _____

Phone _____ Cell phone _____

Email _____

Days & times I'm available. . . _____

Please check how you would like to help:

☐ Patient caregiver

☐ Ride to appointments
(please circle my car or yours)   Other:

☐ Cook meals   ☐

☐ Do laundry   ☐

☐ Clean house   ☐

☐ Run errands   ☐

☐ Grocery shop   ☐

☐ Babysit kids   ☐

☐ Drive kids   ☐

VOLUNTEERS

If there's anything I can do. . .

Name _____

Address _____

Phone _____ Cell phone _____

Email _____

Days & times I'm available. . . _____

Please check how you would like to help:

☐ Patient caregiver

☐ Ride to appointments
(please circle my car or yours)   Other:

☐ Cook meals   ☐

☐ Do laundry   ☐

☐ Clean house   ☐

☐ Run errands   ☐

☐ Grocery shop   ☐

☐ Babysit kids   ☐

☐ Drive kids   ☐

VOLUNTEERS

If there's anything I can do. . .

Name _____

Address _____

Phone _____ Cell phone _____

Email _____

Days & times I'm available. . . _____

Please check how you would like to help:

☐ Patient caregiver

☐ Ride to appointments
  (please circle my car or yours)   Other:

☐ Cook meals   ☐

☐ Do laundry   ☐

☐ Clean house   ☐

☐ Run errands   ☐

☐ Grocery shop   ☐

☐ Babysit kids   ☐

☐ Drive kids   ☐

VOLUNTEERS

If there's anything I can do. . .

Name _____

Address _____

Phone _____ Cell phone _____

Email _____

Days & times I'm available. . . _____

Please check how you would like to help:

☐ Patient caregiver

☐ Ride to appointments
   (please circle my car or yours)   Other:

☐ Cook meals   ☐

☐ Do laundry   ☐

☐ Clean house   ☐

☐ Run errands   ☐

☐ Grocery shop   ☐

☐ Babysit kids   ☐

☐ Drive kids   ☐

VOLUNTEERS

If there's anything I can do. . .

Name _____

Address _____

Phone _____ Cell phone _____

Email _____

Days & times I'm available. . . _____

Please check how you would like to help:

☐ Patient caregiver

☐ Ride to appointments
(please circle my car or yours)   Other:

☐ Cook meals   ☐

☐ Do laundry   ☐

☐ Clean house   ☐

☐ Run errands   ☐

☐ Grocery shop   ☐

☐ Babysit kids   ☐

☐ Drive kids   ☐

VOLUNTEERS

If there's anything I can do. . .

Name _____

Address _____

Phone _____ Cell phone _____

Email _____

Days & times I'm available. . . _____

Please check how you would like to help:

☐ Patient caregiver

☐ Ride to appointments
(please circle my car or yours)   Other:

☐ Cook meals   ☐

☐ Do laundry   ☐

☐ Clean house   ☐

☐ Run errands   ☐

☐ Grocery shop   ☐

☐ Babysit kids   ☐

☐ Drive kids   ☐

VOLUNTEERS

If there's anything I can do. . .

Name _____

Address _____

Phone _____ Cell phone _____

Email _____

Days & times I'm available. . . _____

Please check how you would like to help:

☐ Patient caregiver

☐ Ride to appointments
     (please circle my car or yours)   Other:

☐ Cook meals   ☐

☐ Do laundry   ☐

☐ Clean house   ☐

☐ Run errands   ☐

☐ Grocery shop   ☐

☐ Babysit kids   ☐

☐ Drive kids   ☐

VOLUNTEERS

If there's anything I can do. . .

Name _____

Address _____

Phone _____ Cell phone _____

Email _____

Days & times I'm available. . . _____

Please check how you would like to help:

☐ Patient caregiver

☐ Ride to appointments
(please circle my car or yours)   Other:

☐ Cook meals   ☐

☐ Do laundry   ☐

☐ Clean house   ☐

☐ Run errands   ☐

☐ Grocery shop   ☐

☐ Babysit kids   ☐

☐ Drive kids   ☐

If there's anything I can do. . .

Name _____

Address _____

Phone _____ Cell phone _____

Email _____

Days & times I'm available. . . _____

Please check how you would like to help:

☐ Patient caregiver

☐ Ride to appointments
(please circle my car or yours)   Other:

☐ Cook meals   ☐

☐ Do laundry   ☐

☐ Clean house   ☐

☐ Run errands   ☐

☐ Grocery shop   ☐

☐ Babysit kids   ☐

☐ Drive kids   ☐

If there's anything I can do. . .

Name _____

Address _____

Phone _____ Cell phone _____

Email _____

Days & times I'm available. . . _____

Please check how you would like to help:

☐ Patient caregiver

☐ Ride to appointments
   (please circle my car or yours)   Other:

☐ Cook meals   ☐

☐ Do laundry   ☐

☐ Clean house   ☐

☐ Run errands   ☐

☐ Grocery shop   ☐

☐ Babysit kids   ☐

☐ Drive kids   ☐

VOLUNTEERS

If there's anything I can do. . .

Name _____

Address _____

Phone _____ Cell phone _____

Email _____

Days & times I'm available. . . _____

Please check how you would like to help:

☐ Patient caregiver

☐ Ride to appointments
(please circle my car or yours)   Other:

☐ Cook meals   ☐

☐ Do laundry   ☐

☐ Clean house   ☐

☐ Run errands   ☐

☐ Grocery shop   ☐

☐ Babysit kids   ☐

☐ Drive kids   ☐

VOLUNTEERS

If there's anything I can do...

Name _____

Address _____

Phone _____ Cell phone _____

Email _____

Days & times I'm available... _____

Please check how you would like to help:

☐ Patient caregiver

☐ Ride to appointments
   (please circle my car or yours)   Other:

☐ Cook meals   ☐

☐ Do laundry   ☐

☐ Clean house   ☐

☐ Run errands   ☐

☐ Grocery shop   ☐

☐ Babysit kids   ☐

☐ Drive kids   ☐

VOLUNTEERS

If there's anything I can do. . .

Name   _____

Address   _____

Phone   _____   Cell phone   _____

Email   _____

Days & times I'm available. . .   _____

Please check how you would like to help:

☐   Patient caregiver

☐   Ride to appointments
     (please circle my car or yours)   Other:

☐   Cook meals   ☐

☐   Do laundry   ☐

☐   Clean house   ☐

☐   Run errands   ☐

☐   Grocery shop   ☐

☐   Babysit kids   ☐

☐   Drive kids   ☐

VOLUNTEERS

If there's anything I can do. . .

Name _____

Address _____

Phone _____ Cell phone _____

Email _____

Days & times I'm available. . . _____

Please check how you would like to help:

☐ Patient caregiver

☐ Ride to appointments
(please circle my car or yours)   Other:

☐ Cook meals   ☐

☐ Do laundry   ☐

☐ Clean house   ☐

☐ Run errands   ☐

☐ Grocery shop   ☐

☐ Babysit kids   ☐

☐ Drive kids   ☐

If there's anything I can do. . .

Name _____

Address _____

Phone _____ Cell phone _____

Email _____

Days & times I'm available. . . _____

Please check how you would like to help:

☐ Patient caregiver

☐ Ride to appointments
(please circle my car or yours)   Other:

☐ Cook meals   ☐

☐ Do laundry   ☐

☐ Clean house   ☐

☐ Run errands   ☐

☐ Grocery shop   ☐

☐ Babysit kids   ☐

☐ Drive kids   ☐

There is no exercise better for the heart than reaching down and lifting people up.
— John Andrew Holmes Jr.

Notes

_____

_____

_____

_____

_____

_____

_____

_____

_____

_____

_____

_____

_____

Notes

Notes

Notes

PART FOUR

JOURNAL

Journal

In the book of life, the answers aren't in the back.
— Charlie Brown

Journal

_____

_____

_____

_____

_____

_____

_____

_____

_____

_____

_____

_____

_____

Journal

Journal

Journal

Journal

Journal

_____

_____

_____

_____

_____

_____

_____

_____

_____

_____

_____

_____

_____

Journal

Journal

Journal

Journal

Journal

Journal

Journal

Journal

_____

_____

_____

_____

_____

_____

_____

_____

_____

_____

_____

_____

_____

_____

Journal

Journal

_____

_____

_____

_____

_____

_____

_____

_____

_____

_____

_____

_____

_____

_____

Journal

Journal

Journal

Journal

Journal

Journal

Journal

Journal

_____

_____

_____

_____

_____

_____

_____

_____

_____

_____

_____

_____

Journal

Journal

_____

_____

_____

_____

_____

_____

_____

_____

_____

_____

_____

_____

_____

_____

Journal

Journal

_____

_____

_____

_____

_____

_____

_____

_____

_____

_____

_____

_____

_____

Journal

Journal

_____

_____

_____

_____

_____

_____

_____

_____

_____

_____

_____

_____

_____

Journal

Journal

Journal

Journal

Journal

Journal

Journal

Journal

_____

_____

_____

_____

_____

_____

_____

_____

_____

_____

_____

_____

_____

Journal

Journal

Journal

Journal

_____

_____

_____

_____

_____

_____

_____

_____

_____

_____

_____

_____

_____

Journal

Journal

Journal

_____

_____

_____

_____

_____

_____

_____

_____

_____

_____

_____

_____

Journal

Journal

Journal

Journal

Journal

_____

_____

_____

_____

_____

_____

_____

_____

_____

_____

_____

_____

_____

Journal

Journal

_____

_____

_____

_____

_____

_____

_____

_____

_____

_____

_____

_____

Journal

Journal

Journal

Journal

_____

_____

_____

_____

_____

_____

_____

_____

_____

_____

_____

_____

_____

Journal

Journal

Journal

Journal

Journal

Journal

Journal

_____

_____

_____

_____

_____

_____

_____

_____

_____

_____

_____

_____

_____

Journal

Journal

Journal